I0774945

Optimal Prostate Wellness

A Comprehensive Guide to prevent cancer and enhance Prostate Health Naturally

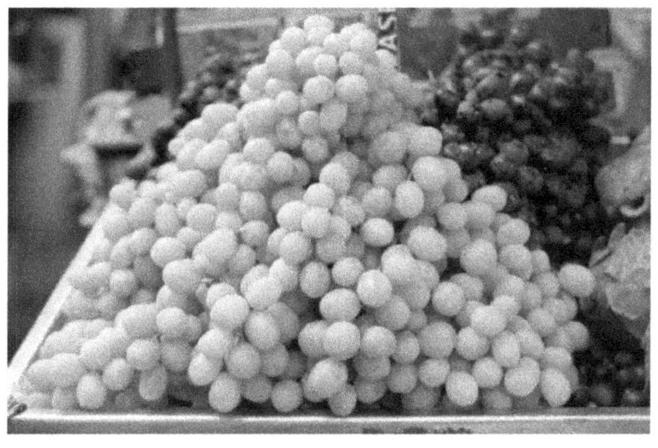

Healthy Happy Me

Copyright © 2024 by Healthy Happy Me

All rights reserved. No part of this book may be reproduced in any form or by any electronic or mechanical means, including information storage and retrieval systems, without permission in writing from the publisher, except by a reviewer, who may quote brief passages in a review.

Although every precaution has been taken to verify the accuracy of the information contained in this book, the author and publisher assume no responsibility for any errors or omissions. No liability is assumed for the damages incurred from the use of the information contained within.

Table of Contents

Introduction

Let me introduce you to Eriggs, a respected sixty-year-old man who is well-regarded in the community for having created a profitable company over the years and is now retiring with grace. A peaceful morning found Eriggs sitting under the shady oak tree in his backyard, thinking about ways to improve the health of his prostate and get over the news that he had prostate cancer, which he had gotten the day before at his regular check-up. Eriggs found solace in the doctor's straightforward methods, which gave him hope that a treatment was possible, even if he was sure that such a diagnosis would bring about fear. His hope? To conquer prostate cancer and enjoy his golden years of retirement with his family.

Over the course of his therapy, Eriggs came to terms with the necessity of giving up certain lifestyle choices that were harmful to his health. He pledged to improve the quality of his diet, exercise regularly, and take medication as prescribed. This change evolved into a comprehensive project with the dual goals of improving his general prostate health and combating prostate cancer.

Eriggs is a key role model in the book "Optimal Prostate Wellness: A Comprehensive Guide to Prevent Cancer and Enhance Prostate Health Naturally," where he demonstrates the steps that need to be taken to both prevent and treat prostate health problems. Supported by insights from the World Cancer Research Fund International, which defines Prostate cancer as the second most commonly occurring disease in males and the fourth most prevalent cancer worldwide, this book encourages you to join us on a journey of learning. Together, we will navigate the complexities of the prostate, identify common health issues related to the prostate, and investigate natural therapies that improve prostate health and guard against prostate cancer. The narrative also explores dietary and lifestyle changes designed to promote prostate health.

Come explore with us and enjoy the path to the best possible prostate well-being. Enjoy!

Understanding Prostate Health
Importance of Proactive Measures

For all men, understanding the nuances of prostate health is essential. On this journey, we explore the prostate's critical role in both sexual health and reproduction. The walnut-sized gland, located directly below the bladder, grows continuously during the early stages of adulthood and is controlled by testosterone levels that decrease with aging. It protects sperm viability and facilitates urethral closure by aiding in the generation of seminal fluid during ejaculation.

The relationship between testosterone and an abnormal growth of the prostate gland highlights the delicate balance of testosterone. As testosterone levels fall, the prostate's enzymes transform more of this hormone into dihydrotestosterone (DHT), which plays a major role in prostate growth and the development of several prostate disorders.

Understanding the risk factors is essential for preserving prostate health, necessitating preventative action. The significance of dietary decisions is highlighted by the fact that obesity is identified as a primary cause of prostate cancer and associated problems. It is advised to replace animal fats with plant-based sources like nuts and avocados and to cut back on dairy consumption. When combined with consistent exercise, these lifestyle changes help maintain a healthier prostate.

Preventive care also means regular check-ups at the doctor, where tests for Prostate-Specific Antigen (PSA) and testosterone become critical in older men. This all-encompassing strategy protects the prostate from future health issues and builds its resilience.

Crucially, this investigation into prostate health is a call to action as much as an evaluation. Through the ensuing chapters, we will uncover natural solutions and practical takeaways, culminating in an all-inclusive manual for naturally preventing cancer and improving prostate health.

Chapter One

Prostate Health Fundamentals
Anatomy and Function of the Prostate Gland

Like the liver and kidney, the prostate gland is an essential auxiliary organ in the male reproductive system. A thorough knowledge of the anatomy of the prostate is essential because it establishes the link between abnormalities in the structure and function of this vital gland and a variety of prostate health issues.

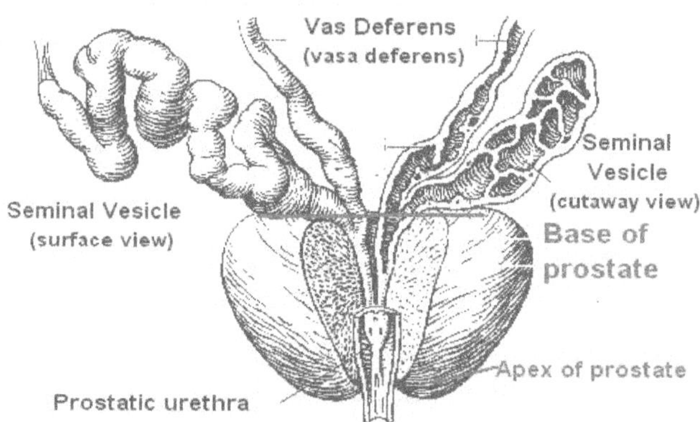

Source:
National Cancer Institute - SEER Training Modules. (n.d.). Prostate Cancer: Anatomy. Retrieved [November 28, 2023], from https://training.seer.cancer.gov/prostate/anatomy/

Overview of the Prostate Gland

Located above the deep perineal pouch (UGD) and behind the neck of the bladder, the prostate gland is an essential part of the male reproductive system. Located in front of the lowest third of the rectum and behind the lower portion of the symphysis pubis, its precise position emphasizes its critical function.

The urogenital diaphragm, or deep perineal pouch, acts as a structural border at the apex of the bladder, while the **urethra** and **ejaculatory duct** puncture its base. The posterior side borders the bottom section of the rectum, and the anterior side borders the **retropubic area** and **puboprostatic ligament.** The middle rectal artery and inferior vesicle support the arterial supply, while the levator ani (levator prostate) flanks the sides.

When we examine the internal structure of the prostate, the urethra, ejaculatory duct, and prostatic utricle are the three main parts that stand out. Together, these components support the gland's complex operation.

Five lobes make up the prostate gland, and each has unique qualities.

1. **Anterior Lobe:** With no glands, this lobe has a special function in the construction of the prostate.

2. **Posterior Lobe:** This lobe, which is behind the urethra and ejaculatory duct, is essential to the gland's general operation.

3. **Middle Lobe:** This lobe is characterized by a high gland density and may become obstructed, which could have negative health effects.

4. **The right lobe:** A lateral element that adds to the overall symmetry.

5. **Left Lobe:** This lobe's counterpart, the right lobe, completes the bilateral makeup.

The prostate's structural integrity is supported by the layers of protection around it:

1. **Fibrous Capsule**: This outer layer, which encircles the gland, is vital for support.

2. **Fibrous Sheath (Pelvic Fascia):** This layer, which encircles the fibrous capsule, houses the prostatic venous plexus, an essential part of the vascular supply.

3. **Rectoprostatic Fascia:** This layer protects the prostate from surrounding anatomical tissues by acting as a barrier against the rectum.

Gaining an understanding of the prostate's complex location, internal structures, and protective layers is essential to understanding its function and possible health consequences. This synopsis paves the way for a more in-depth investigation of prostate health and its relationship to structural anomalies within this vital gland.

Role in Reproductive Health
1. **Secretion of Prostatic (Seminal) Fluid:**

The prostate gland secretes prostatic (seminal) fluid, which is alkaline in nature. This fluid contains acid phosphatase, a proteolytic enzyme that plays a crucial role in preventing sperm from clumping together. This action ensures that sperm are ready for effective penetration of the egg. It's important to note that elevated levels of acid phosphatase can be indicative of conditions such as prostate cancer, often associated with the obstruction of the ducts of the glands. The primary function of prostatic fluid is to nourish and support sperm, contributing to the overall composition of semen.

2. **Production of Prostaglandin**:

In addition to prostatic fluid, the prostate gland secretes prostaglandin. Prostaglandins are hormone-like substances that serve various physiological functions, including the regulation of inflammation and smooth muscle contraction. In the context of the prostate, prostaglandins may play a role in the contraction of smooth muscles within the gland, contributing to the expulsion of semen during ejaculation. The specific functions of prostaglandins in the prostate are complex and may involve multiple physiological processes.

Other functions include:

3. **Influence on Urinary Function**: The position of the prostate, which encircles the urethra, may affect how well the bladder functions. Benign prostatic hyperplasia, or

BPH, is a disorder in which the prostate gland grows larger with age. This enlargement can put pressure on the urethra, causing symptoms like poor urine flow, difficulty urinating, and increased frequency of urination.

4. **Prostate-Specific Antigen (PSA) Secretion**: The bloodstream is exposed to a protein produced by the prostate gland known as prostate-specific antigen (PSA). Elevated PSA levels may be a sign of prostate cancer, infection, or inflammation. PSA is a regularly used measure for prostate health.

Common Prostate Health issues

The prostate gland, an essential part of the male reproductive system, is prone to several health problems. For early detection and suitable medical management, understanding these disorders is essential.

1. Benign Prostatic Hyperplasia (BPH):

BPH, or benign prostatic hyperplasia, is a common aging condition for men. The urethra may get blocked as a result of pressure from the growing prostate. The symptoms include painful ejaculation, poor urine flow, frequent urination (particularly at night), difficulties starting a pee, and stiffness or pain in the lower back, hips, pelvis, or rectal area. Although BPH is not malignant, it can have a major negative influence on one's quality of life and ability to urinate.

2. **Prostate inflammation (also known as prostatitis):** Bacterial infections or other causes may contribute to prostatitis, which is an inflammation of the prostate gland. It can cause symptoms including pelvic pain or discomfort, lower back pain, groin pain, penis tip pain, painful urination, and occasionally flu-like symptoms. Acute bacterial prostatitis, chronic bacterial prostatitis, chronic pelvic pain syndrome, and asymptomatic inflammatory prostatitis are the four disorders that fall under the umbrella of prostatitis.

For males under 50, prostatitis is the most prevalent urinary tract problem; for men over 50, it is the third most common.

3. Prostate Cancer:

As the second most frequent cancer in males, prostate cancer is one of the most common diseases to affect men. In the early stages, it may not show any symptoms and often progresses slowly. As people age, their risk increases considerably, especially for those over 50.

Other risk variables consist of:

Age: The risk is higher for men over 50.

Obesity: Studies indicate a link between a heavier weight and a higher risk of prostate cancer.

Race: The prevalence is higher among African American, Native American, and Caribbean men of African heritage and Hispanic men; the percentages are lower among Asian men.

Family History: Although it raises the probability of a diagnosis, a family history of prostate cancer does not guarantee one.

Diet: Eating a diet heavy in fat can increase the risk of prostate cancer.

When symptoms do arise, they may include erectile dysfunction, pelvic or lower back pain, blood in the urine or semen, and trouble urinating. To diagnose prostate cancer in its early stages, when treatment is most successful, routine screenings, such as PSA tests and digital rectal exams, are crucial.

4. UTIs, or urinary tract infections:

Urinary tract infections can impact the prostate gland, resulting in symptoms including burning or pain when urinating, urgency, and frequent urination. Antibiotic therapy must be started as soon as possible to stop the infection from spreading.

Men should make routine check-ups and screenings a priority, especially as they get older, to monitor the health of their prostates and identify any potential problems early. Obtaining timely medical guidance is important for accurate diagnosis and treatment of any worrisome symptoms.

Chapter Two

Factors Affecting Prostate Health

Hormones, choices regarding lifestyles, environmental circumstances, diet and nutrition, and other factors interact intricately to determine prostate health. It is essential to comprehend how these factors affect the prostate to promote general health and reduce the risk of problems related to the prostate.

Knowing the underlying causes of prostate health concerns is essential because, if appropriately managed, these factors can either have a favorable or negative effect on prostate health.

Diet and Nutrition

i. **High-Fat Diet:** Eating a diet high in fat has been linked to a higher risk of health problems relating to the prostate, such as prostate cancer. Prostate health can be improved by reducing saturated fat intake and consuming a well-rounded, nutrient-rich diet full of fruits, vegetables, and whole grains.

ii. **Antioxidants and Vitamins:** Several antioxidants, like tomato-derived lycopene, and vitamins, including vitamin E, have been connected to possible advantages for prostate health. These vital elements can be obtained by including foods like leafy greens, tomatoes, berries, nuts, and almonds in the diet.

Not only are diet and nutrition important for overall health, but they are also important for keeping the prostate healthy. Making wise dietary decisions can help maintain prostate health and reduce any dangers related to particular foods or beverages.

Lifestyle and Exercise

i. **Physical Activity**: Studies have demonstrated the beneficial effects of regular exercise on prostate health. It supports general cardiovascular health in addition to lowering the risk of obesity-related problems and helping people maintain a healthy weight. Jogging, brisk walking, and other aerobic exercises are examples of activities that can promote prostate health.

ii. **Maintaining a Healthy Weight**: Prostate cancer and other disorders related to the prostate are known to be exacerbated by obesity. Maintaining a healthy weight and reducing the risk of prostate health problems can be achieved by implementing a balanced diet and regular physical activity.

Environmental Influences

i. **Exposure to Chemicals**: Prostate health problems, including prostate cancer, have been related to several environmental factors, including exposure to certain chemicals. Prostate cancer risk may be increased by occupations that expose workers to combustion byproducts (firefighters, for example) or agricultural pesticides (farmers, for example).

ii. **Lifestyle**: Adopting unhealthy behaviors like smoking and excessive drinking might be detrimental to the health of the prostate. In particular, smoking has been associated with a higher risk of prostate cancer that is aggressive. Reducing alcohol consumption and quitting smoking are two healthy behaviors that can improve prostate health.

Understanding the effects of the environment is essential. Some occupations may expose workers to substances that could be harmful to their prostate health. When these environmental elements are understood, pre-emptive steps to minimize risk can be taken.

Hormonal Balance

Impact of Hormones on Prostate Health

The intricate interaction between androgens and estrogens within the prostate gland sheds insight into the complicated topic of hormones and prostate health. In terms of prostate biology, steroid hormones are significant. Dihydrotestosterone (DHT) and testosterone are the two androgens that are most prevalent in men. Dihydrotestosterone is produced from testosterone by the enzyme 5-alpha reductase. Prostate cancer growth and initiation have long been associated with androgens in particular. Notably, a key component of the treatment of prostate cancer has been androgen ablation therapy (AAT), which targets androgenic hormones. Early treatments used estrogen-based strategies, but these were abandoned because of serious cardiovascular side effects.

The use of luteinizing hormone-releasing hormone (LHRH) agonists or antagonists in AAT methods has developed over time, but its effectiveness is limited and patients frequently relapse, eventually reaching an androgen-independent condition. Interestingly, the role of estrogens, derived from androgens, has been underestimated. Both local paracrine effects that specifically target the prostate tissue and systemic endocrine effects that indirectly reduce androgens are exhibited by estrogens.

By comprehending these processes, systemic therapy may give birth to more specialized and efficient treatments. For example, blocking the enzyme aromatase, which changes androgens into estrogens, has been investigated, but because estrogen signaling involves many receptor subtypes (ERα and ERβ), the results have been inconclusive.

The prostate is affected by estrogen in several ways. They exhibit anti-proliferative properties and cause aberrant proliferation in the basal layer, which results in squamous metaplasia. Prostate inflammation has been linked to estrogens, mainly through ERα, but ERβ may have anti-inflammatory properties. Both androgens and estrogens are required for carcinogenesis, but they are not sufficient on their own to cause cancer.

As the disease progresses, ERβ's expression changes, making its function in suppressing prostatic cancer unclear. Nonetheless, research indicates that ERβ activation may possess anti-carcinogenic characteristics. Maintaining prostate health appears to depend on the balance of AR, ERα, and ERβ activities.

In conclusion, even if androgens are important in prostate health and disease, knowing how complex estrogens may be, especially about ERα and ERβ, opens up new possibilities for more specialized and possibly successful treatments. Using the subtleties of estrogen receptor activity to target therapies may be possible, but there are still obstacles to overcome before this knowledge can be applied in clinical settings, particularly about the many ways that ERβ is expressed at different stages of prostate disease.

Strategies for Hormonal Balance

The complex relationship between hormonal dynamics and prostate health is shown by the way that hormone balance and health interact inside male physiology. The harmful effects of hormone dysregulation on the prostate are significant, and the delicate balance between testosterone and estrogen becomes critical. Specifically, imbalances in hormone levels, such as an overabundance of estrogen or a shortage of testosterone, cause the development of benign prostatic hyperplasia (BPH), which highlights the significance of preserving a balanced hormonal system.

A crucial component of proactive intervention is the early detection of the subtle indicators of hormone imbalance. The symptoms are warning signs that demand close monitoring of hormone balance, and they include everything from widespread weariness and decreased libido to erratic mood swings and unexplained weight gain. To prevent potential prostate problems, quick and focused actions must be initiated based on the recognition of these symptoms.

The mutually beneficial relationship between a well-planned diet and regular exercise becomes apparent while maintaining a balanced hormonal environment. A healthy diet that is well-rounded and rich in nutrients essential for hormone regulation, along with a regimen of consistent exercise, plays a crucial role in coordinating hormone balance and, in turn, in promoting prostate health.

1. **Testosterone Regulation:** The introduction of compounded testosterone gels has brought about a significant transformation in the conventional view of testosterone regulation. Its innovative methodology offers a sophisticated way to maintain testosterone levels in the ideal mid-to-upper range. The criticality of accurate dosage in conjunction with the necessity of patient education forms the foundation for effectively controlling testosterone levels and strengthening the defenses of prostate health.

2. **Estradiol Control:** Another area of customized hormone regulation is estradiol regulation by customized aromatase inhibitor drugs, such as letrozole or anastrozole. Specifically designed for male physiology, these lower-dose versions provide a focused approach to address estradiol abnormalities that might be early signs of prostate-related diseases.

3. **Nutritional Support:** Nutraceuticals, such as zinc, selenium, vitamin D, and omega-3 fatty acids, are the peak of nutrition and go beyond traditional dietary guidelines. Their many functions, which include inhibiting 5α-reductase, which is involved in the conversion of testosterone, and exhibiting anti-inflammatory properties, portend advantages for the prostate's overall health.

4. **Stress Management:** A complex approach to stress management is required due to the widespread impact that stress has on hormonal homeostasis. By reducing the disruptive effects of stress on hormonal homeostasis, the integration of cutting-edge stress-reduction techniques

like yoga and meditation emerges as a proactive tool positively influencing prostate health.

5. **Youthful Hormonal Levels:** It is worth noting that preserving youthful hormone levels represents a paradigm shift in the way that optimal prostate health is approached. Maintaining testosterone, estradiol, and dihydrotestosterone levels similar to those in adolescence plays a critical role, highlighting the long-term importance of hormonal balance in reducing the latent risks from prostate disorders throughout life.

All told, the tactics discussed outline a broad range of interventions, including pharmaceutical advancements, nutraceutical supplements, and maintaining young hormone levels. It is critical to recognize that each person's response is unique and requires customized advice from medical experts. Research is still in its early stages, but it is expected to reveal more subtleties and deepen our knowledge of these tactics in the ever-changing field of prostate health. Hormonal dysregulation could be a hidden danger to prostate health, but a well-planned combination of certain supplements and lifestyle changes could strengthen a stronghold of prostate health.

Chapter Three

Natural Remedies and Prevention Strategies

Herbal Supplements and Their Effect

In America, around one-third of men utilize complementary therapies, such as herbal supplements, to manage prostate disorders. Although research indicates that there may be some advantages to treating prostate cancer, care must be taken because there may be drug interactions. Herbs like St. John's wort, for example, might influence the liver enzymes that break down medications, which can alter how effective they are.

Certain supplements may increase bleeding risks when used with drugs like aspirin or anticoagulants. Examples of these supplements were palmetto for enlarged prostates and melatonin for possible slowing of cancer progression. It's unclear, nevertheless, if these supplements actually increase prostate cancer or serve as a true preventive measure.

Supplements containing beta-sitosterol and African cherry have demonstrated efficacy in treating prostate cancer. The FDA has not, however, given these supplements treatment approval.

The noteworthy SELECT trial examined the effect of vitamin E and selenium supplementation on the risk of prostate cancer. Men who took vitamin E exhibited a surprisingly 17% higher risk than those who took a placebo. Furthermore, excessive vitamin E or selenium dosages showed little benefit and occasionally even caused harm, particularly to individuals with pre-existing elevated selenium levels.

To put it simply, herbal supplements aren't magic fixes. Even though they might help some men, it's important to make an informed decision and speak with a doctor before using them in treatment or preventative strategies for prostate disorders.

Dietary Modifications for Prostate Health

Establishing a healthy eating pattern can help preserve the prostate by preventing prostate-related illnesses and minimizing symptoms. Diet is important for the general health of the body, and the prostate is no different. Fruits and vegetables should always be a part of a diet.

Prostate-Friendly Foods

1. **Lycopene-containing fruits:**

Red pigment lycopene, which is present in a variety of fruits, has demonstrated encouraging effects in lowering the incidence of prostate cancer and enlargement.

Tomatoes (particularly those with high levels), watermelon, grapefruit, papaya, and apricots are sources of lycopene.

2. **Fish Oil and Fish:**

Omega-3 fatty acid-rich fish and fish oil are good for overall health but there is conflicting information about their effect on cancer risk.

Omega-3 Fatty Acid Sources: Mackerel and Salmon

3. **Citrus Fruits:** Citrus fruits, which are rich in vitamin C, have been linked to a lower incidence of prostate cancer.

Vitamin C-rich foods include oranges, lemons, and grapefruit.

4. **Nuts Rich in Zinc**: Nuts high in zinc, such as almonds, peanuts, and cashews, have been shown to have a beneficial impact on lowering the prostate size and prostate cancer risk.

5. **Brazil Nuts**: Brazil nuts, which are high in selenium, help lower the incidence of prostate cancer.

6. **Vitamin D:** Taking supplements or salmon is a good way to get vitamin D, which has been associated with a lower incidence of benign prostatic hyperplasia.

7. **Beta-Sitosterol**: This substance, which is present in dark chocolate, avocados, pistachios, saw palmetto, Pygeum, peanuts, rice bran, wheat germ, soybeans, corn oils, stinging nettles, and canola oil, enhances the flow of urine in people who have enlarged prostates. It has been discovered that beta-sitosterol helps BPH. Beta-sitosterol cannot be converted to testosterone in contrast to cholesterol

8. **Allium Vegetables:** Adding onions and garlic to your diet can lower your risk of benign prostatic hyperplasia.

Including a range of these items in your diet can help maintain the health of your prostate and lower your chance of enlargement and related issues. As always, get individualized advice from a healthcare expert.

Vitamins and Minerals for Optimal Function

1. **Vitamin D:**

Function: Essential for immune system control, bone health, and the prevention of chronic illnesses.

Prostate Focus: Associated with a lower incidence of prostate cancer and enlargement of the prostate.

Source: While getting outside in the sun is beneficial, you should also eat foods high in vitamin D, such as fatty fish, egg yolks, and fortified foods.

2. **Vitamin E:**

Advantages: Promotes better blood flow, hormone balance, and anti-inflammatory and antioxidant effects.

Support for the Prostate: demonstrated to lower inflammation and may impede the development of an enlarged prostate.

Natural sources include leafy greens, nuts, and seeds.

3. **Vitamin C:** Promotes the synthesis of collagen and has strong anti-inflammatory and antioxidant properties.

Prostate Effect: Promotes the health of the prostate gland, counteracts free radicals, and helps to minimize inflammation.

Food sources: present in a variety of fruits and vegetables, including bell peppers, oranges, strawberries, kiwis, and broccoli.

4. **Vitamin B6:** Impacts: Supports neurotransmitter activity, controls hormones, and shrinks the prostate.

Benefits for the Prostate: Good at easing the symptoms of an enlarged prostate in the urine.

Fish, poultry, avocados, potatoes, and fortified cereals are examples of food sources.

5. **Zinc:** The Protective Mineral Roles: has anti-inflammatory qualities, prevents the conversion of testosterone, and causes prostate cell death.

Prostate Support: Research indicates that taking supplements can help reduce symptoms of BPH and decrease an enlarged prostate.

Sources: A necessary mineral that can be found in a variety of foods, such as dairy, almonds, and meat.

6. **Saw palmetto:** The herbal relief compounds contain anti-inflammatory and anti-androgenic properties. **Prostate Support:** This may help reduce inflammation, lower DHT levels, and protect the prostate from oxidative stress. **Forms:** Available in capsules, tablets, and liquid extracts.

Including these vitamins and minerals in your diet or thinking about supplements under medical advice may help maintain a healthy prostate. Keep in mind, that a balanced and nutritious diet is the best defense against oxidative stress.

Exercise and Its Impact on Prostate Health

Despite the relatively little attention it has received in the study, regular physical activity turns out to be a critical component in supporting prostate health. Although there aren't many studies that explicitly examine how exercise affects this walnut-sized gland, what is known about its potential advantages is persuasive.

Research emphasizes the use of exercise as a therapeutic intervention for a range of disorders connected to the prostate, such as prostate cancer, benign prostatic hyperplasia (BPH), and prostatitis. Remarkably, results from the continuing Harvard Health Professionals Follow-up Study show a significant correlation between a higher level of physical exercise and a lower risk of developing BPH. Even low- to moderate-intensity activities, such as regular walking at a moderate pace, demonstrate tangible benefits for prostate health.

Through the use of males with chronic prostatitis in a randomized controlled experiment, Italian researchers increased our understanding of this condition. Compared to a non-aerobic exercise group, the group that participated in aerobic exercises—brisk walking three times a week—reported less anxiety and sadness, less prostatitis pain, and an overall increase in their quality of life.

A study involving more than 1,400 men found that exercise affects prostate cancer which is still in the early stages. Those who walked vigorously for at least three hours each week showed an astounding 57% decreased risk of cancer progression in comparison to their less active peers.

Stressing the value of regularity, a comprehensive workout regimen that includes at least 30 minutes of physical activity most days of the week shows promise as a means of preserving prostate health. But before starting an exercise program, it's important to speak with a healthcare provider, just like you would with any lifestyle modification. Your physician can offer you specific advice and assist you in creating a program that suits your current state of health and level of fitness.

In summary, it is impossible to overlook the positive relationship between prostate health and regular physical exercise. We take preventative measures to ensure the health of this essential organ by exercising regularly and consulting medical professionals.

Chapter Four

Mind-Body Connection and Prostate Health

Stress Management Techniques

Deep breathing exercises, yoga, and mindfulness meditation are some of the techniques that can help lower stress levels and ease the symptoms of Benign Prostatic Hyperplasia (BPH). Managing stress is crucial for preserving prostate health.

Meditation and Prostate Health

The ability of meditation, an effective technique for enhancing mental and emotional health, to promote physical health is becoming more widely acknowledged. This guided meditation, designed with prostate health in mind, blends mindfulness practices with visualization to provide a restorative and therapeutic atmosphere. This extensive note examines the relationship between prostate health and meditation, outlining the steps of guided meditation and its possible effects on prostate health.

With its ability to induce a state of peace and relaxation, meditation is a powerful technique for boosting overall well-being.

Worries and stress make it difficult for the body to heal. By reducing these influences, meditation helps to create the ideal setting for recovery.

Preparation for Meditation:

- Switch off your phone and remove any distractions from the area before starting the meditation.
- You can choose to meditate while seated or while lying down, depending on how comfortable and relaxed you want to feel.
- To improve the overall quality of the meditative experience, it is stressed how important it is to loosen and relax the limbs.

Pay Attention to Your Breath:

- The first stage in mindfulness meditation is to focus on your breathing.

- By concentrating on the breath, one can induce mental tranquility and stillness by slowing down the flow of thoughts.

Breathing in Peace:

- Participants are instructed to see the energy they exhale as a soothing, bright blue color.
- Breathing in this blue energy represents breathing in serenity; expelling signifies letting go of any pent-up tension or bad energy.

Progressive Relaxation:

- Next, the body is gradually relaxed, beginning at the head and working down to the toes.
- The soothing blue light envelops every bodily part, encouraging deep relaxation.

Targeted Healing for the Prostate:

- Focus moves to the prostate region, where the blue energy changes to a red light that is warm and healing.

- It is imagined that the red light penetrates deeply into each prostate cell, repairing and cleaning it.

Creation of a Healing Energy Circle:

- To improve the flow of healing energy, the individual creates a circle with their thumbs and first fingers.
- As this circle widens, a red fluorescent light surrounds the entire body, focusing on aches and pains and encouraging deep healing.

Space Visualization:

- As part of the meditation, the participant visualizes themselves in space, surrounded by stars and a crystal-clear waterfall.
- Warm water floating beneath the space waterfall purifies the entire body, concentrating especially on the prostate.

Re-entering the Present:

As the meditation comes to a gentle end, participants are invited to progressively open their eyes while feeling completely at ease within.

Intentional breathing, mindfulness, and visualization techniques are all used in this guided meditation to produce a comprehensive experience that supports prostate health. Through cultivating a profound state of tranquility and facilitating the flow of restorative energy, this meditation gives people a tool to enhance their general well-being. Frequent practice may enhance not only your mental well-being but also the prostate's health and vitality.

Mindfulness and Relaxation Techniques

A comprehensive strategy that incorporates yoga, mindfulness, and relaxation techniques is proving to be an effective ally in the quest for optimal prostate health. By cultivating an attentive awareness of the present moment, mindfulness as a practice enables people to participate in daily activities with acceptance and nonjudgmental curiosity. With the right instruction, such as recorded sessions and guided sessions, this practice can be improved and the groundwork for improved wellbeing can be laid.

Understanding mindfulness tenets, workings, and real-world applications is all part of the training. People can learn experiences-spanning skills from this training, such as appreciating the flavor and aroma of food when eating. Numerous advantages of mindfulness techniques are demonstrated by research, especially for men with prostate cancer. These benefits include a decrease in symptoms of worry and despair as well as a reduction in fears about the recurrence of cancer.

A study headed by Professor Victorson shows that the transformational power of mindfulness goes beyond the regimented programs. Following an eight-week mindfulness session, men on Active Surveillance for prostate cancer experienced long-lasting gains. Positive improvements following traumatic events persisted for up to 12 months, while reductions in anxiety persisted for up to 6 months and reductions in uncertainty for up to 12 months. The participants reported gains in their interpersonal skills and a strengthening of their character.

Men's stated improvements following mindfulness training include:

1. **Better Emotional Regulation**:

- "I've been able to develop a clearer, more honest relationship with my thoughts as a result of the stress reduction."
- "I step back and observe and then adjust. I experience my feelings but don't always act on them."

2. **An Increase in Self-Awareness**:

- "I'm able to handle stress better now that I'm more relaxed and aware."
- "The breathing exercises have helped me become more aware of my thoughts and feelings, allowing me to react to situations in a more positive way."

3. Increased Tolerance and Patience:

- "I am more understanding of other people's eccentricities."
- "I have become more patient and tolerant of myself."

5. Living More in the Now:

- "I am living more in the now, with less gratitude, anxiety, and closeness to my partner."
- "I am more mindful, more in the moment."

6. Greater Appreciation:

- "I am more appreciative of the goodness of people."
- "I am thankful for every day."

7. Relationship Enhancement:

- "I am less combative, more laid back, and I pay attention to what other people have to say."
- "I'm nicer to my wife and tell her more I love her."
- "I consider before I act. I'll deal with my emotions as quickly as possible. I'll talk more about my thoughts and feelings with my wife."

As technology advances, online mindfulness courses provide customized curricula that address the special needs and worries of cancer patients, especially those with prostate cancer. These programs are effective in lowering cancer-related exhaustion, boosting general quality of life, and improving mental health outcomes. Beyond the limitations of location, online programs offer the privacy needed to finish sessions on their own and the option to participate whenever it is most convenient. Online mindfulness classes provide an accessible way for people to seek support at any point along their cancer journey, from diagnosis to treatment and survivorship, as the number of men with prostate cancer climbs.

In conclusion, combining yoga, mindfulness, and relaxation methods results in a synergistic strategy for prostate health that is ideal. Through the practice of mindfulness, awareness-building, and the incorporation of yoga's physical benefits, people can take a revolutionary step toward improved health and support for their prostate health goals.

Yoga for Optimal Prostate Health

With this carefully chosen series of energizing yoga positions, take the first steps toward prostate health transformation. As you move fluidly through the following postures, cultivate an awareness of the relationship between your body and breath:

1. Vajrasana (The Iron pose): Start with this potent stance, which is recognized to have certain health benefits for the prostate. Vajrasana, or the "Iron Pose," is a basic yoga pose in which you sit on your heels with your knees bent and your lower legs tucked under your thighs. The Sanskrit terms "Vajra," which means thunderbolt or diamond, and "Asana," which means position or posture, are combined to form the name "Vajrasana". Vajrasana combined is sometimes translated as the "Diamond Pose" or the "Thunderbolt Pose." Allow the position to guide you into a calm state of self-awareness while it works its therapeutic power.

Vajrasana can be practiced as follows:

1. Begin by bending down on the floor so that your thighs are parallel to the floor.

2. Plant the tops of your feet on the mat, bringing your knees together and pointing your toes backward.

3. Sit on the folded legs and lower your hips onto your heels.

4. Place your hands on your knees with your palms facing down while maintaining a straight spine and relaxed shoulders.

5. Shut your eyes gently and concentrate on your breathing.

Vajrasana is a popular meditative pose that can be utilized for a variety of purposes, such as breathing exercises, meditation, and preparing for other asanas. It has a reputation for enhancing digestion, supporting the lower back, and enhancing focus.

Among the benefits of Vajrasana are:

1. **Digestive Health:** By enhancing blood circulation in the abdomen area and supporting the operation of the digestive organs, Vajrasana helps facilitate digestion.

2. **Improved Posture:** Vajrasana practice regularly contributes to improved posture by keeping the spine straight and aligned.

3. **Meditation:** Vajrasana is a great pose for meditation because it helps you feel grounded and steady, which helps you focus and become peaceful.

4. **Reduced Stress:** Vajrasana is a simple, calming pose that can help lessen tension and anxiety.

5. **Strengthening Muscles:** The lower back, legs, and thighs are all strengthened by this pose.

It is noteworthy that anyone with knee or ankle problems may find Vajrasana inappropriate. It's best to seek advice from a yoga instructor or other healthcare provider if you experience any discomfort or health issues when doing this pose. To guarantee a secure and comfortable practice, always pay attention to your body and adjust your pose as necessary.

2. **Butterfly Pose**:

Lift your chest, close your eyes, and join the soles of your feet. This is a particularly powerful pose for men; to increase its influence, softly shake your legs.

3. **Janusirsasan:**

- Extend your legs and bend your right leg inward toward your body.
- Take a breath and raise your chest; release it as you progressively bend forward to massage your perineum and lower abdomen.

4. **Paschimottanasana:**

- Reach for your toes with both legs extended.
- As you exhale, keep your back straight and softly bend forward, allowing each breath to lead you further into the stretch.

5. **Purvotasana (Backbend):**

- Take a breath and raise your head and hips to create a powerful stretch for prostate enlargement.
- Gently release your breath again.

6. **Crocodile Pose (Makrasana):**

- Lie on your abdomen with your hands piled on top of one another.
- Take a breath, raise your head, and tilt it to the side.

7. **Ardhbhujangasana (Half Cobra):**

- Stand up gently, placing your palms shoulder-width apart and standing on your elbows.
- Maintain a forward-facing gaze, shoulders down, and chest raised.

8. **Dhanurasana (Bow Pose):**

- Lower your forehead to the floor as you exhale.
- Take a deep breath and raise your head, shoulders, and chest to nourish your back.

9. **Crocodile Pose (Makrasana):**

- Return to the pose with your hands stacked and your face resting comfortably on your head.

10. Wind-Relieving Pose (Pawanmuktasana):

- With each exhale, extend your legs, bend your knees, and bring your forehead to your knees.

11. Lower Spine Twist (Udrakarsanasana):

- To ensure a mild stretch, twist your lower spine by lowering both knees to each side alternately.

12. Half Bridge Pose, or Setubandhasana:

- Inhale, elevating your hips; use your hands or interlocked fingers to support your back.
- Release the posture by exhaling.

13. Savasana (Corpse Pose):

- Spread your legs wide and let your body unwind fully.
- Consider how these poses improve your overall health and support the health of your prostate.

Turn to your right, sit quietly, and enjoy the peace and comfort that surround you to finish the session. Warmth should be felt in your lower abdomen as you gently open your eyes and let the healing energy fill you.

Recall to approach these poses mindfully, and if you have any specific health issues, think about speaking with a medical expert or yoga instructor. Have fun on your path to health!

Psychological Factors in Prostate Health

Although physiological factors are predominantly linked to prostate health, psychological factors may also have an indirect impact. Though they might not be the main cause of prostate problems, psychological variables can improve general health and may have an indirect effect on prostate health.

Men who are receiving treatment for prostate cancer frequently feel a variety of feelings, such as anxiety, despair, exhaustion, and a general feeling of being overwhelmed. These mental health problems have the potential to spread, affecting different facets of a man's functioning. Relationships, especially those with spouses, may be challenging, and financial concerns can become a major source of stress. The experience becomes even more emotionally difficult due to the dread of potential discrimination from employers.

Some potentially pertinent psychological aspects are included below:

1. Mental Health: Conditions such as depression and anxiety can be detrimental to general health. Immune system performance and overall health depend on maintaining mental wellness.

2. Lifestyle Decisions: Stress, anxiety, and depression are examples of psychological variables that might affect lifestyle decisions. Persistent stress may impair the body's defenses against infections and erode the immune system, which may affect prostate health.

For instance, those who are under a lot of stress could be more likely to engage in harmful habits like smoking, eating poorly, or exercising seldom, all of which have an indirect negative impact on prostate health.

3. **Sexual Health:** Prostate health may be indirectly impacted by maintaining a healthy sexual function, since psychological issues may also play a part in sexual health.

4. **Sleep Quality:** Sleep quality has a direct impact on psychological health. Insomnia and irregular sleep habits can have a detrimental effect on the immune system, which may affect prostate health.

5. **Coping Mechanisms:** General health can be impacted by an individual's capacity to manage stress and obstacles in life. Ineffective coping strategies can result in bad behaviors, whilst effective coping strategies can influence improved lifestyle decisions.

6. **Mind-Body Connection**: The mind-body connection is a complex interplay in which psychological variables can affect the immune system and hormone regulation, which may affect several physical functions, including those linked to the health of the prostate.

While psychological aspects can positively impact one's general health and well-being, it's crucial to remember that they are only one facet of the many variables that affect prostate health. Prostate health requires regular exercise, a balanced diet, and regular check-ups with the doctor.

Chapter Five

Medical Approaches and Integrative Solutions

Screening Tests and Early Detection

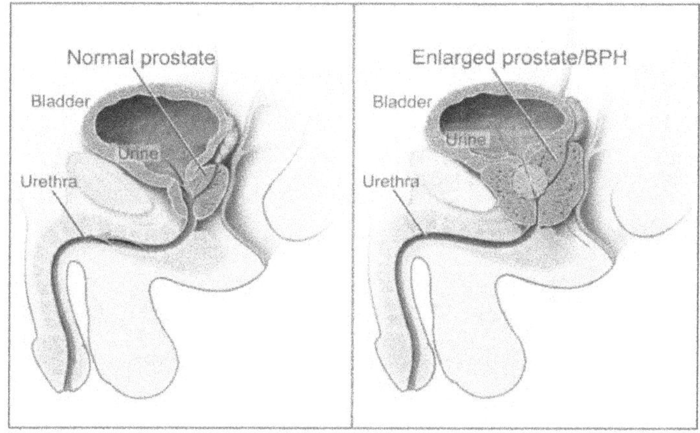

Importance of Regular Check-ups

Routine examinations are essential for preserving the best possible prostate health and general well-being. Regular examinations are essential for the early identification, prevention, and prompt treatment of problems connected to the prostate, including prostate cancer, which is the most common type of cancer in males.

Early identification of prostate cancer is one of the main benefits of routine check-ups. When this cancer is first developing, it frequently shows no signs at all. Healthcare providers can spot anomalies or early indicators of prostate cancer with thorough screenings that include digital rectal exams (DRE) and blood testing for the prostate-specific antigen (PSA). Regular checkups are essential for protecting men's health since they increase the chance of successful treatment and improve long-term outcomes. This is demonstrated by the significant impact early diagnosis has on these outcomes.

These examinations are essential in preventing several prostate-related disorders in addition to detecting cancer. Medical professionals can evaluate the prostate gland's general health and spot any indications of swelling, infection, or inflammation. Early detection of these disorders enables prompt therapies, averting more consequences and preserving ideal prostate health. Regular check-ups are important as a proactive step to promote long-term well-being because of their preventive nature.

Furthermore, by taking care of a variety of prostate-related issues, routine examinations enhance general well-being. Exams like these are used by medical experts to talk about and address issues like changes in urine habits, sexual dysfunction, and urinary difficulties. Patients can receive the right advice, treatment, or referrals to specialists if needed by addressing these issues as soon as possible. During prostate exams, this all-encompassing approach to prostate health makes sure that men address a wider range of problems that could affect their quality of life in addition to possible cancer concerns.

To sum up, scheduling routine examinations is critical to preserving prostate health. These tests have a major positive impact on general health by facilitating the early detection of prostate cancer and helping to prevent several illnesses related to the prostate. Men who take the initiative to schedule routine checkups are proactively protecting their health, encouraging a healthy prostate, and guaranteeing their long-term well-being.

Understanding Screening Tests
What to anticipate from a prostate examination

Patients can anticipate a thorough assessment of their prostate health during a prostate check-up. A physical examination, a review of medical history, and diagnostic testing are usually part of the check-up.

1. Physical Examination: A crucial step in any prostate check-up, the physical examination involves the healthcare provider evaluating the size, shape, and texture of the prostate gland. One common method used in this examination is the digital rectal examination (DRE), which entails inserting a gloved, lubricated finger into the rectum to feel the prostate gland. While this may sound uncomfortable, the procedure is relatively quick and painless, and the medical professional will gently press against the rectal wall to assess the prostate's size, consistency, and any irregularities.

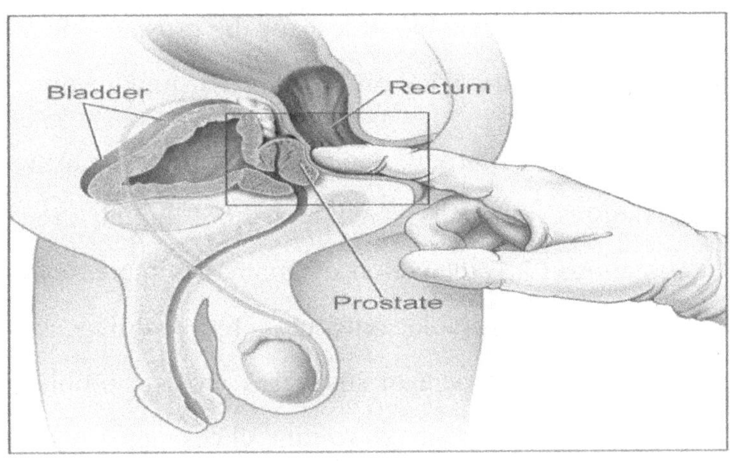

When looking for abnormalities in the prostate, the DRE is essential. It makes it possible for the medical professional to spot any lumps, nodules, or hard spots that can point to the existence of prostate disorders such as benign prostatic hyperplasia (BPH) or prostate cancer. The physician can learn a great deal about the state of the prostate gland by palpating it directly.

It is crucial to understand that the DRE is not a conclusive test for diagnosing diseases of the prostate. Nonetheless, it functions as a preliminary screening instrument that may stimulate additional inquiries if anomalies are identified. The doctor may suggest further testing, such as a prostate biopsy or a blood test for the prostate-specific antigen (PSA) if the DRE reveals any alarming results.

Prostate health is largely dependent on routine physical examinations, which include the digital rectal examination. Early detection of anomalies increases the likelihood of favorable outcomes by enabling rapid diagnosis and treatment of suspected prostate problems. Men should therefore make routine check-ups a priority and never be reluctant to raise any worries or symptoms with their healthcare professional.

2. Review of Medical History

Examining the patient's medical history is a crucial step in a prostate checkup. This is an important stage because it gives the healthcare professional an understanding of the patient's general health and helps them discover any illnesses or risk factors that could affect the patient's prostate health.

The healthcare provider can obtain information regarding past medical conditions, surgeries, drugs, and lifestyle choices that may have an impact on the prostate by reviewing the patient's medical history. Diabetes, heart disease, and obesity are a few illnesses that have been connected to a higher risk of prostate issues. The medical professional can evaluate the patient's prostate health by taking these conditions into account if they are aware of them.

Prostate health is also significantly influenced by family history. Genetics can play a role in prostate disorders, such as prostate cancer. Prostate difficulties may increase the likelihood of acquiring similar problems if close relatives, like a father or brother, have experienced them. The medical professional can ascertain whether the patient has a higher risk and may require more regular or specialized screenings by looking over the family history.

In conclusion, it is critical to go over the patient's medical history during a prostate examination to comprehend general health status and identify potential risk factors for prostate health. It enables medical professionals to take into account past illnesses, prescription drugs, and lifestyle choices that may affect the prostate. In addition, evaluating the family history aids in identifying any hereditary susceptibility to prostate issues. Healthcare professionals can offer appropriate screenings and individualized therapy to support prostate health by obtaining this information.

3. Diagnostic Examinations

Several diagnostic tests may be carried out to evaluate the prostate gland's health during a prostate check-up. These tests assist in locating any anomalies or possible indications of problems related to the prostate. **The prostate-specific antigen (PSA)** test is one of the most widely used procedures.

The PSA test quantifies the blood's concentration of PSA, a protein secreted by the prostate gland. Prostate cancer and other illnesses may be indicated by elevated PSA readings. It is crucial to remember that raised PSA levels can also be caused by other conditions, thus having a high PSA level does not always indicate prostate cancer.

A transrectal ultrasound is another imaging modality that is frequently employed during a prostate examination (TRUS). A little probe is inserted into the rectum during this procedure to take pictures of the prostate gland. When looking for anomalies like tumors or enlarged prostates, TRUS can be helpful.

To assess the prostate further, imaging methods like as computed tomography (CT) scans and magnetic resonance imaging (MRI) may be employed in addition to PSA tests and TRUS. The prostate gland and associated tissues can be seen in great detail thanks to these imaging modalities, which aid in the diagnosis and staging of prostate diseases.

All things considered, the diagnostic procedures carried out during a prostate examination are essential for determining the prostate gland's state of health and identifying any possible problems.

Urine testing is an additional procedure that can be used to look for anomalies or indicators of illness.

Recommendations for Scheduling Check-Ups

Some practical principles should be followed when arranging routine check-ups for prostate health to guarantee consistency and adherence to specified intervals.

1. **Age and Risk Factors:** Taking into account your age and risk factors is the first step in arranging check-ups. In general, men who are older than 50 ought to have routine prostate exams. However, it's best to begin screening earlier, around age 45, if you have a family history of prostate cancer or other risk factors like being African-American.

2. **Consultation with Healthcare practitioner**: Depending on your unique health state, it is essential to discuss the right frequency of check-ups with your healthcare practitioner. To determine the best interval, your doctor will take into account several criteria, including your medical history, current symptoms, and general state of health.

3. **Adhere to Screening criteria:** Medical groups like the American Cancer Society and the U.S. Preventive Services Task Force have established screening criteria that must be followed. Based on age and risk factors, these guidelines specify the suggested timeframes for digital rectal exams (DRE) and prostate-specific antigen (PSA) testing.

4. **Regularity and Consistency:** When it comes to making check-up appointments, consistency is essential. It's critical to follow the suggested intervals and to keep all scheduled appointments on time. Frequent examinations enable the early identification of any possible problems and prompt intervention where necessary.

5. **Keep a Health journal:** You may stay on top of your check-up schedule and avoid missing any appointments by keeping a health notebook. Make a note of the dates of your prior check-ups and schedule follow-up appointments.

By adhering to these recommendations and scheduling routine examinations, you can proactively preserve the health of your prostate and identify any possible issues early on.

Early Intervention's Advantages

Men who take early action to improve their prostate health can benefit greatly. Early prostate problem detection makes it possible to start treatment on time and achieve better results. The following are some main advantages of early intervention:

1. **A higher likelihood of successful treatment:** Less intrusive and more effective treatment alternatives are frequently available for prostate issues that are discovered early. As a result, there may be a greater chance of controlling the illness and stopping it from getting worse.

2. **Better quality of life:** Prostate health issues can be promptly managed with early care, which can help reduce symptoms and enhance general well-being. Men can encounter fewer difficulties and have greater physical and emotional health by treating the issue early on.

3. **Decreased chance of complications:** Prostate disorders can result in complications like sexual dysfunction, urinary issues, and even prostate cancer if they are not addressed. Better long-term results and reduced risk of these problems can be achieved with early detection and treatment.

4. **Peace of mind:** Men who get regular checkups and early intervention may rest easy knowing that their prostate health is being watched after and that any possible problems are being dealt with right away. This proactive strategy can support general well-being and reduce anxiety.

In summary, routine check-ups and early intervention in prostate health are critical. It has many advantages, such as better quality of life, lower risk of complications, higher likelihood of a good outcome, and peace of mind.

Treatment for prostate cancer, which affects around one in seven men and is the leading cause of cancer-related deaths in Western nations, must be comprehensive and multidisciplinary. This section clarifies advanced prostate cancer and offers a holistic plan that combines traditional therapies with cutting-edge methods, with a focus on the use of insulin-sensitizing drugs.

1. **Primary Treatments for Localized Disease:** Radiation therapy or radical prostatectomy are the first lines of defense against quickly progressing localized prostate cancer, with success rates well over 90% in both cases.

2. **The Difficulties of Androgen-Deprivation Therapy (ADT):**

Growth and survival of prostate cancers are mostly dependent on androgen signaling.

After a median amount of time, castrate-resistant prostate cancer (CRPC) results from ADT's disruption of androgen production through the use of LHRH agonists or antagonists.

Due to the past lack of viable treatment options for CRPC, there has been a strong focus on developing novel medicines that target the androgen axis.

3. **Obesity and Prostate Cancer:** Obesity increases the risk of prostate cancer by three times, and there is a close correlation between the two conditions as the population ages.

The acceleration of CRPC in the presence of obesity and ADT-induced hyperinsulinemia highlights the critical need to treat this metabolic factor.

4. **Insulin-Reducing Treatments as Possible Supplements:**

This section emphasizes the possible relevance of currently available insulin-lowering medicines in light of the function that hyperinsulinemia plays in the course of CRPC.

These treatments, which are well-established in the context of type 2 diabetes and the metabolic consequences of obesity, show promise as adjuvant medicines for the treatment of prostate cancer.

5. **Clinical Implications and the Need for Integration**: This factor is currently disregarded in the usual treatment of prostate cancer, despite the higher risk of cardiovascular and cancer-related mortality linked to ADT-induced hyperinsulinemia.

The current wave of studies and clinical trials seeks to clarify the advantages of using anti-insulin therapy in addition to established and novel treatments for prostate cancer.

To sum up, this section's integrative approach recognizes the complexity of prostate cancer and aims to maximize treatment outcomes by fusing traditional treatments with cutting-edge tactics. The focus on logical justification for insulin-sensitizing drugs represents a paradigm change in the management of the metabolic components of prostate cancer progression. Anti-insulin therapy integration has the potential to improve the general health of patients with prostate cancer and increase the effectiveness of treatments currently being researched and tested by the medical community.

Chapter Six

Case Studies and Success Stories

Join renowned urologist and prostate cancer specialist Dr. Michael Turner as he takes you on a moving journey through the struggles and victories endured by men with the disease. In addition to treating prostate cancer, Dr. Turner, who oversees the Urology Department at St. Andrews Medical Center, was personally diagnosed with the disease in 2005. His distinct viewpoint clarifies the emotional rollercoaster that patients go through as well as the crucial part that medical professionals play in influencing their cancer journey.

The diagnosis of prostate cancer thrusts Dr. Turner into the patient-doctor relationship from the opposite side. His struggle unravels the emotional complexities that patients face—fear, uncertainty, and the drive to overcome the hurdles of prostate cancer.

For patients, the day they are diagnosed with prostate cancer is a moment in time stuck in place. The unbelief, the bizarre nature of the diagnosis, and the consuming concerns about what lies ahead are all reflected in Dr. Turner's memory. Through a variety of patient experiences, this universal experience is examined, highlighting the emotional impact of the initial diagnosis.

As with other cancers, there are social stigmas associated with prostate cancer that prevent honest conversations. A common struggle for men is their unwillingness to discuss their illness. Breaking the silence of addressing patients' hopes, worries, and anxieties with healthcare providers and their support networks is something that Dr. Turner emphasizes as being crucial.

Throughout the prostate cancer journey, effective communication and individualized care become essential elements. Patients of Dr. Turner emphasize how important it is to have a healthcare professional who is not only clinically skilled but also empathetic and eager to meet with them on a personal level to build trust and a feeling of support.

One common theme is the blessing of having a physician who supports their patient during their prostate cancer journey. The notion that the doctor-patient connection is based on a partnership based on a common determination to defeat prostate cancer is further supported by Dr. Turner's dedication to being a caring companion.

The personal account of Dr. Michael Turner and the accompanying testimonies from patients highlights the life-changing nature of a prostate cancer diagnosis. These stories highlight how important it is for healthcare professionals to provide clinical expertise, compassion, and steadfast support. By exploring these stories, we seek to encourage and uplift those who are dealing with prostate cancer by showing that the path can be accomplished with courage, resiliency, and optimism if one has the proper support system and an empathetic healthcare provider.

Case One

Starting a new chapter in the face of prostate cancer before the age of 50 is a rare trip, but that's exactly what occurred to James in 2015. James, who was diagnosed with localized prostate cancer at the age of 48, discusses what it was like to be diagnosed, how he dealt with health professionals about his sexuality, how he began a new relationship, and how he included holistic approaches into his treatment.

Being Diagnosed

James discovered blood in his pee one day. Since it had only happened twice, he didn't give it much thought and simply attributed it to stress or drinking too much alcohol. He eventually gave his local sexual health clinic a call, and that same day, he saw a general practitioner. He was directed to a urologist at Blackpool Victoria Hospital after talking about his symptoms. James underwent many scans and a blood test to determine the nature of the issue.

After that, he got a letter stating that an urgent biopsy was required. His mind was racing over this, which was highly concerning. He recalls asking himself a variety of questions, such as "Am I going to die?"

James was pleased with how quickly everything was completed after receiving a prompt appointment for a biopsy. Upon returning for his results, the consultant was quite straightforward. He looked at the screen and made notes before saying, "You have prostate cancer." James was then presented with an enormous number of options and information, but he was unable to comprehend or think for himself. He was taken aback. He went from knowing nothing about cancer to being diagnosed with it.

Receiving Medical Care

James had two options: radiation or surgery (radical prostatectomy). He was still just 45 years old, and his PSA had increased to 40. He concluded that his best course of action was surgery. James had surgery at the Royal Preston Hospital in June 2016. He was informed following surgery that the cancer could not be completely removed. Additionally, he was informed that the cancer was no longer contained in his prostate as previously believed. It had begun to move towards his gut and bladder. James was advised to undergo intense radiation therapy for 32 weeks as a result. He additionally had hormone therapy. The news was disheartening, and there were moments when he did ask himself, "Why me?"

James looked into holistic alternatives to supplement conventional treatment for his cancer. Considering the possible benefits of herbs and lifestyle alterations for overall well-being, incorporating them into his routine became imperative. Though it was difficult, James discovered that maintaining an optimistic outlook was beneficial. Cancer is not something that anyone chooses, so if you have it, you just have to deal with it. He continued working since it seemed to divert attention from him. Some may argue that's not feasible, but for James, being employed helped. Having a break is beneficial while dealing with cancer daily.

Holistic Approaches to Treatment

James adopted all-encompassing strategies to enhance his overall health. He included herbal supplements that have been linked to improved cancer management; nonetheless, he always consulted his medical team before introducing any new regimen. To support general health, he also implemented lifestyle changes like a balanced diet, consistent exercise, and mindfulness exercises.

Talking about Sexuality to Health Professionals

James has never come out as gay to a medical professional, but he is upfront about who he is. His sexuality was never brought up, and no one ever questioned him about it. However, his interactions with hospital workers were mainly positive. The questions he asked made the majority of medical experts aware of his sexual orientation.

He would advise being upfront, honest, and open about one's identity. He would also advise disclosing whether one is gay or bisexual because the way these identities are handled and treated can vary greatly. All of it comes down to your strength and character.

Starting a New Relationship During Treatment

When James was first diagnosed, he didn't have a partner; instead, he relied on his mother for support for the majority of his appointments and the help of other family members and friends. However, he enjoyed being alone himself. It was vital to him to have room to think things through and sort everything out in his head. He knew support was there if he needed it.

While undergoing radiotherapy, he first connected with his spouse online. Although James was anxious to see him in person, he was open about his treatment and any adverse effects, such as erectile difficulties. From the beginning, his spouse showed great understanding and support. These days, sex is different, and when things don't work out as planned, especially in a new relationship, it can be discouraging. However, life is more than just sex, and you don't have to push yourself or force it. It matters more if you have a solid and loving connection since it is what matters most in life.

Now that they're married, James's spouse goes to his doctor's appointments with him. They've had positive experiences together, and he's always been accepted and included in his care. He poses inquiries that James would never consider. This has been very beneficial.

In Manchester, James also goes to the Out With Prostate Cancer Support group. He no longer lives apart from the group. Now, his spouse goes to gatherings with him and participates in discussions. In the group, discussions are focused on what members want to know and no topic is off-limits. To help new members make better decisions for themselves, James now feels equipped to speak candidly with them about his experience, his story, how things have affected his body, and the holistic methods that have improved his well-being.

Case 2

Jake Anderson's account of his January 2010 struggle with stage three prostate cancer was an emotional rollercoaster, with me doubting the reason behind everything and having periods of "why me?" wondering what I could have done to deserve this.

Along with 37 rounds of radiation therapy, I underwent hormone therapy. They were concerned about possible risks, so surgery was not an option. Thus, the choice was made to treat it and leave it alone. The actual treatment just took two minutes, but well, the preparation was a whole afternoon affair. I would be measured for the treatment, and each time I would have to lie in the same position. Strangely enough, they took longer to check that I was positioned correctly than actually giving me the treatment.

Then the side effects set in: fatigue, irritability, and indifference. It struck me hard, but I felt fortunate. The radiographer even remarked I performed quite well. The acute need to use the restroom—a significant side effect of the radiation therapy—was one of the hardest things I had to deal with. Since I had no control over it, I had to carefully arrange my outings and make sure I was near restrooms.

On some days, the exhaustion was so great that the idea of going to radiotherapy felt like an enormous undertaking. What, nevertheless, kept me going? My incredible brother-in-law Every single day, he would follow along and encourage me by saying, "36 down, 35 to go." Up until the last session, we adhered to that regimen, using his triumphant phrase, "One down, none to go," to climb those steps. We decided it was time for a celebration and went across the street to the bar for a well-earned beer.

Granted, there are still occasions when I'm too tired to go out, but I still attempt. The secret is to remain positive at all times—100% and even more so. That's the attitude you need to have if you want to defeat something. It has been a road, but perseverance and optimism have been invaluable.

Chapter Seven

Further Concepts

Collaborating with Healthcare Professionals

Improving prostate health and tackling the issues related to prostate cancer require close collaboration with medical professionals. One excellent program that encourages health professionals to investigate new models of care for men with prostate cancer is Prostate Cancer UK's Health and Social Care Professionals program.

Even though the program is no longer in operation, its influence is still great. Through its financing of 59 healthcare professionals in a range of healthcare institutions, including the NHS, Prostate Cancer UK has enabled 44 different projects to be implemented. Over 38,000 people's lives have been positively impacted by these programs, which provide care and support in primary and secondary healthcare settings across the United Kingdom.

The program's success serves as a reminder of how crucial it is for healthcare providers and prostate health organizations to work together. Improved patient outcomes and experiences are made possible by these collaborations, which make it possible to create and test innovative care models. A key focus of Prostate Cancer UK's ongoing efforts to improve care delivery is the development of clinical leaders capable of taking on the pressing issues surrounding prostate health.

Working together with healthcare providers on an ongoing basis is still crucial in the changing world of prostate health. We can all work together to promote prostate wellness and the standard of care given to individuals with prostate cancer by encouraging innovation, exchanging knowledge, and encouraging clinical leadership.

Integrating Natural Approaches with Medical Guidance

There are several natural methods that you can combine with medical advice to enhance the health of your prostate. Some easy behavioral adjustments can help reduce the symptoms of enlarged prostate glands that cause problems with urination, according to a Harvard Health article. These include reducing fluid intake before heading out in public or beginning a vacation, waiting one to two hours before drinking anything, peeing as soon as you feel the need, scheduling regular bathroom breaks, and taking your time to fully empty your bladder.

Prostate cancer may also be successfully treated with straightforward measures like green tea, pomegranates, and consistent exercise.

It is crucial to remember that these natural therapies should not be used in place of direct medical counsel from your doctor or other licensed healthcare provider; rather, they should be used in addition to medical advice.

Building a Proactive Healthcare Team

Having a strong team of specialists to guide your health is essential for developing a proactive healthcare team for prostate health. It's important to use a multidisciplinary team approach and the assistance of numerous experts and qualified healthcare providers when developing a care plan specifically for prostate cancer. This entails obtaining the assistance of multiple specialist physicians as well as other professionals like nurses, dietitians, and mental health counselors.

You should think about adding the following professionals and specialists to your team if you have prostate cancer:

1. **Providers of primary care:** For routine checkups and common issues, you see your PCP, who is typically your family physician. The PSA (prostate-specific antigen) test or DRE (digital rectal exam) that resulted in the diagnosis of prostate cancer may have been conducted by your PCP. To treat symptoms or concerns as they emerge, your PCP will help coordinate all facets of your healthcare team and refer you to subspecialists. This could include

psychological disorders or urological concerns that arose during treatment. Following treatment, your PCP will assist in developing a survivorship care plan for the future and ensuring that it is shared with other members of your team. They'll probably be able to handle a lot of your follow-up exams and assist you in lowering future risk factors like smoking and obesity as well as monitoring for recurrence.

2. **Urologists:** You can be referred to a urologist for additional testing and treatment if you have been diagnosed with prostate cancer or if you suspect it. Prostate cancer is one of the conditions that urologists, who specialize in surgery, address in the male reproductive system and urinary system. Your urologist will help give you treatment options and may perform any surgeries you might need, such as a radical prostatectomy.

3. **Cancer specialists:** A healthcare professional who focuses on treating cancer is called an oncologist. Radiation oncologists and medical oncologists are the two categories of oncologists who might be on your prostate cancer team. Treatment using radiation therapy is the area

of expertise for radiation oncologists. This could involve internal radiation (brachytherapy) or external beam radiation therapy for prostate cancer. Medical oncologists concentrate on alternative drug regimens and cancer treatment alternatives such as hormone therapy and chemotherapy.

If you feel that your needs aren't being addressed, it is acceptable—in fact, it's encouraged—to politely question your healthcare team and confront individuals who are assisting you. But initially, the team must be formed to shape it into precisely what you require.

Maintaining Prostate Health Throughout Life

Aging and Prostate Health

Since the overall number of mutations accumulates over time, aging is linked to an increased risk for the development of most cancer forms. This is true even for prostate cancer cells.

Long-term Strategies for Wellness

1. **Adopt a Mediterranean diet:** Fresh fruits and vegetables, whole grains, legumes, fatty fish, nuts, and seeds are among the foods high in healthy fats found in a Mediterranean diet. It is thought to be the most effective method of maintaining overall prostate health without the use of questionable vitamins or supplements, none of which have been demonstrated to be effective in preventing prostate cancer.

2. **Limit red meat consumption:** Limit your consumption of red meat, including beef, hog, lamb, and goat, and processed meats, such as bologna and hot dogs. Rather, choose lean protein sources including fish, poultry, and plant-based proteins.

3. **Spend some time in the sun:** Prostate health depends on vitamin D. Prostate cancer risk may rise with insufficient sun exposure. On the other hand, sunscreen is essential for shielding your skin from damaging UV radiation.

4. **Engage in regular exercise:** Physical activity helps lower the chance of prostate cancer. Both aerobic and non-aerobic workouts, like leg lifts, sit-ups, and stretching, are beneficial. Examples of aerobic exercises include fast jogging.

5. **Get screened**: Depending on your risk category—high- or average-risk—different screening guidelines exist for prostate cancer. Beginning at age 40, if you belong to a high-risk category, you should think about getting examined for prostate cancer. Between the ages of 45 and 55, men who are at normal risk are recommended to think about getting screened.

Keep in mind that these are only broad recommendations. Seeking individualized guidance and recommendations from a healthcare professional is always the best course of action.

Conclusion

Let's sum up by saying that attaining the best possible prostate wellness requires a thorough awareness of the structure of the prostate as well as a variety of illnesses, natural therapies, and medical procedures. Prostate cancer survivors like Eriggs are resilient, and his story emphasizes the value of preventative care for men's health.

Recap of Key Strategies

Key techniques for maintaining optimal prostate health include regular screening of PSA levels and understanding of signs and symptoms associated with prostate diseases. Men should take an informed and proactive attitude to prostate health, particularly as they get older. Moderate dietary modifications, hormone-balancing techniques, and lifestyle alterations are essential for maintaining prostate well-being. Nonetheless, to guarantee a customized and secure strategy, it is critical to confer with healthcare professionals before implementing any changes.

Moving Forward Towards Optimal Prostate Health

Going forward, the focus should be on combining medical interventions with holistic therapies, like lifestyle changes and natural remedies. The path taken by Eriggs serves as an excellent example of how these tactics can aid in recovery. It serves as a reminder that although medical care is necessary, proactive measures taken to preserve ideal prostate health have a substantial positive impact on general well-being.

To put it simply, the road to ideal prostate health is a peaceful collaboration between patients and their medical professionals. Men can take the first steps towards long-term prostate wellness and well-being by becoming knowledgeable, adopting good lifestyle habits, and consulting a professional.

References

Risbridger, G. P., Ellem, S. J., & McPherson, S. J. (2007). Estrogen action on the prostate gland: a critical mix of endocrine and paracrine signaling. *Journal of Molecular Endocrinology,* 39(3), 183–188. https://doi.org/10.1677/JME-07-0053

3 ways exercise helps the prostate (yes, the prostate) - Harvard Health. https://www.health.harvard.edu/mens-health/3-ways-exercise-helps-the-prostate-yes-the-prostate.

National Cancer Institute (NCI). (n.d.). Prostate Cancer Screening (PDQ®)–Patient Version. Retrieved from https://www.cancer.gov/types/prostate/patient/prostate-screening-pdq

Glossary of Terms

- **The Androgen Receptor (AR):** This is a protein that plays a critical role in mediating the effects of androgen hormones, such as testosterone and dihydrotestosterone (DHT), within the prostate gland. It's essential for the normal development, function, and growth of the prostate. The AR interacts with androgens, regulating gene expression and influencing various processes, including prostate cell growth and differentiation.

- **Urologist:** A medical professional specializing in the diagnosis and treatment of conditions related to the urinary tract and male reproductive system.

- **Yoga Asana:** A specific posture or pose in yoga practice that involves physical and mental discipline. Certain yoga asanas, such as pelvic-focused poses, may contribute to prostate wellness by promoting flexibility, blood circulation, and relaxation.

- **Lycopene:** A carotenoid antioxidant found in tomatoes and other red fruits, believed to have prostate health benefits.

- **Mindfulness Meditation:** A practice that focuses on being present in the moment, potentially beneficial for overall well-being.

- **Hormone Therapy:** Medical treatment involving the manipulation of hormones, sometimes used in prostate cancer management.

www.ingramcontent.com/pod-product-compliance
Lightning Source LLC
Chambersburg PA
CBHW071609270726
48661CB00019B/1765